Two Wolf Taijiquan

All Rights Reserved

Copyright©2015 Cody Toye

Published by Ink Blood Publishing
~~*

Table of Contents

About Two Wolf Taijiquan

The Name:

The name was taken from the Cherokee tale "The Wolves Within" it is as follows:

An old grandfather said to his grandson, who came to him with anger at a friend who had done him an injustice.

"Let me tell you a story. I too at times have felt a great hate for those that have taken so much, with no sorrow for what they have done. But hate wears you down, and does not hurt your enemy. It is like taking poison and wishing your enemy would die. I have struggled with these feelings many times."

He continued

"It is as if there are two wolves inside me. One is good and does no harm. He lives in harmony with all around him and does not take offense when no offense was intended. He will only fight when it is right to do so and in the right way. But the other one, ah!

He is full of anger. The littlest thing will set him into a fit of rage. He fights everyone, all the time, for no reason. He cannot think because his anger and hate is so great. It is helpless anger, for his anger will change nothing. Sometimes, It is hard to live with these two wolves inside me, for both of them try to dominate my spirit."

The boy looked intently into his grandfather's eyes and asked

"Which one wins grandfather?"

The grandfather smiled and quietly said

"The one you feed"

The Combination and the Origin:

Just like "The Wolves Within", Two Wolf Taijiquan promotes mastering one's self long before hurting others. Just as the tale says,

"He will only fight when it is right to do so and in the right way."

So shall we. For this reason, the system consists mostly of joint locks, ward offs, and basic self- defense.

We will fight in the right way, we shall not completely destroy someone for the minor offense of a flying fist driven by anger alone.

During my travels overseas, I landed in the nice little town of Germiston in the Gauteng Province of South Africa. While there, a group of local children seen a minor display of my martial arts and asked for a lesson. Needing the exercise and practice and always willing to help out children I happily agreed.

I started with different basic techniques from the Tracy System of Kenpo. Before I knew it, I found myself teaching a whole class of children ranging from eight years of age to eighteen.

As time went by, I started adding Yang Style Tai Chi, teaching the form and techniques to some of the older kids and Pencak Silat to the middle aged children.

Something was missing. I started feeling odd about teaching such impressionable children some of the brutal tactics found in both Kenpo and Silat. I glossed over the arm breaks, disregarded the harsh take downs and knife fighting techniques.

This was where the two wolves battled inside me for a moment. Do I change such effective techniques that are proven to work so well? Do I only teach joint locks, blocks, and forms?

The answer came to me. I shall combine the internal concepts of Tai Chi with the effective less brutal techniques. The result will be a sincere and effective self-defense system that allows you to escape with your life without damaging another's.

Two Wolf Taijiquan is South Africa's Tai Chi system.

The Form

The form is made up of *fifty* movements that combine Kenpo, Silat, and Yang Taijiquan. It flows together keeping the original internal concepts of Tai chi; yet it hides the movements of several techniques within it. This allows the practitioner to utilize muscle memory when practicing the techniques. This guide is meant for instructors, practitioners; both current and prospective; as a tool. It is not meant to be utilized alone, only to help one practice what they have learned hands on. For this reason, I will use key words while describing movements and techniques.

Starting with your legs slightly apart and knees gently bent, place both arms slightly in front palms down.

- Rise
- Sink
- Rise
- Sink
- Single Whip Left Side into Wing Break Left Side
- Single Whip Right Side into Wing Break Right Side
- Inverted Hands like Clouds
- Push
- Water Wheel
- Closing the Gate Left Side
- Hands like Clouds Right side
- Energy Ball Right Knee
- Left step Forward, Condense
- Twirl the Sun
- Energy Ball Right Knee
- Grasping Sparrows Tail
- Roll Back and Push
- Sun Moon Hands
- Energy Ball Left Knee
- Step Forward Right Knee
- Energy Ball Right Knee
- Grasping Sparrows Tail
- Roll Back and Push
- Rise
- Sink

- Outward Cloud Hands
- Inward Cloud Hands
- Outward Cloud Hands
- Hook
- Lock
- Sun Beats Wall Left Side
- Cloud Breaks Wing Left Side
- Step Forward Right Knee
- Sparrow Hits Ground
- Step Forward Left Knee
- Cloud Breaks Wing Left Side
- Step Forward Right Knee
- Sparrow Hits Ground
- Step Back Right Knee
- Sparrow Takes Flight
- Sparrow Hits Ground
- Single Whip Left Side, Wing Break
- Single Whip Right Side
- Step Back Left Foot
- Wing Break Right Side
- Single Whip Left Side
- Delayed Sword
- Repulse Monkey X3
- Lifting The Sun
- Settle the Qi

Tips for a Better Form

When performing the form keep in mind that all rising motions should be accompanied with an inhale and all sinking motions with an exhale. Nice slow deep breaths throughout the form will help bring the Chi from your Dan-Tien to the rest of your body. When creating an energy ball, pay attention to which hand is supposed to be on top. When you look down, your knee should be bent and you should not be able to see your foot. Remember, nice and slow. Practice don't make perfect. Perfect practice makes perfect.

Techniques

- Bear Embraces the Sun (Shoulder Grab)

  {P26}
- Dragon Wields a Mace (Side Grab Right)

  {P27}
- Spitting Cobra (Shirt Grab)

  {P28}
- Chickens Talon (One Hand Wrist Grab)

  {P29}
- Water Collides With Cliff (Double Wrist Grab)

  {P30}
- Evading the Sun (overhead Club)

  {P31}
- Breaking the Cloud (Punch)

  {P32}
- Catching the Koi (Punch)

  {P33}
- Monkey Brushes Its Hair (Punch)

  {P34}
- Monkey Dance (Back Grab)

  {P35}
- Repulse Monkey (Punch)

  {P36}
- Twirling the Sun (Punch)

  {P37}

- Enter Dan-Tien (Hammer Lock)
- Gorilla Weaves Basket (Two Hand Shirt Grab)
- Sword Strikes Sparrows Wing (Punch) A.B.
- The Five Gorillas (Punch)
- Lion Strikes Prey (Punch) Lap Sao Drill
- The Snake and the Dart (Triple Punch)
- Yin Yang Sun (Straight Across Wrist Grab)
- Hammer Strikes Anvil (One Hand Shirt Grab)

Step by Step

~~*

Inward Cloud Hands

From the neutral position; an opponent will throw a punch. (Mostly practiced against right punches, since the majority of the population is dominantly right handed).

You will come up your center-line with your left hand, blocking from the inside; turning your hips. Your right hand will come up your center-line and catch the arm close to the elbow, turning your hips the opposite way. This will result in a joint lock of their right arm.

Outward Cloud Hands

From the neutral position; an opponent will throw a right punch. You come up your center-line turning your hip's, you catch the punch with your right hand from the outside. Coming up your center-line and turning your hips, your left hand will sweep through the fold of your opponent's elbow, resulting in a gentle repel or throw.

Repelling the Cloud

Essentially, this technique has the same setup as "Outward Cloud Hands". You will still turn your hips and catch the punch from the outside with your right hand. You will bring the opponents arm in a gentle circular motion down your center-line and place your left hand beside your right on their arm. Sinking, you will push in towards them. You want to aim their arm towards their own center-line, pushing and repelling them backwards.

Sun Beats the Wall

Using the same setup as "Repelling the Cloud", you will turn your hips and catch their punch from the outside with the right hand. In a circular motion, you will bring their arm down your center-line. INSTEAD of placing your left hand on their arm beside your right, you will reach across their body with your left hand and place it on the left side of their head and push to the left. This will tip them slightly off balance. Immediately, take your right hand and push on their left shoulder, repelling and pushing your opponent away.

Sparrow Hit's the Ground

From the neutral position, your left hand will guard your face. As the right punch comes in, you will slap the punch from the outside with your left hand and step forward with your left foot. You will immediately grab your opponent's thumb side of the fist with your left hand and your opponent's pinkie side of the fist with your right hand. You will step past them with your right foot (on the outside of their right leg) and twist their hand so that it passes over their shoulder and torques their body. As the name suggests, you want to aim for the ground behind them, making the "Sparrow" or the fingers of their fist, touch the ground.

Sparrow Takes Flight

The exact same setup as "Sparrow Hit's the Ground". Except AFTER you have step pasted them on the right side with your right leg and torque the body, you will immediately step backwards with your right leg and sweep their fist past your right hip, aiming the sparrow first low, then high as it passes you, repelling them or throwing them.

Sparrow Break's Its Wings

From a neutral position, when the punch comes, you will come up your center-line and turn your hips, catching the punch from the outside with your right hand. Stepping forward with your left foot, you will place your left hand on their shoulder blade. Pushing down with your left hand, you will pull with your right, forcing their shoulder to lock and their body to propel towards the ground face first.

Koi Swims Circles

From a neutral position, when the punch comes, you will come up your center-line and turn your hips, catching the punch on the inside with the left hand. Immediately grab your opponent's wrist with the left and grab the bicep with the right. Stepping back with your left foot, you will turn your hip and swing your opponents arm in a circular motion. To do this, think of your opponents arm as a baseball bat and swing in the same fashion. This will result in a repel or a throw.

Single Whip

From a right punch, (taught from either side) your left arm will sling upwards, blocking the punch by connecting with their forearm with the bony prominences of your left wrist. Your fingers and your thumb should be touching each other in a "plum flower fist". Immediately, while your left hand connects with their punch your right hand will shoot straight out and strike their chest in the center with your palm. This will result in a hard push or repel backwards.

Drunken Retreat

From a neutral position, with your left hand in guarding your face; your right arm will come inward in an "L" shape. This will sandwich their arm between your left hand and your right forearm. Leaning backwards as you catch their arm, you will lift your knee and kick straight forward, bearing your weight forward as you do so. You should aim for whichever target is easiest to get too based off your flexibility and body posture. For those who are shorter or have trouble kicking high, aiming for the knee or the groin is preferable. For those who can; a solid kick in the center of the chest will propel them backwards with much force.

Bowing to the Sparrow

This is done against a single handed choke. The beginning of both A and B are the same and it is as follows. Your left hand will grip their thumb side of their hand and your right will grip their pinkie side of their hand. Making a big gesture, you will bow to them while pinning their hand, resulting in a sharp pain from a wrist lock.

A. After bowing and locking their wrist, you will let go of their thumb with your left hand and reach across with your right, gripping their thumb side. Peeling their hand off of your throat, you will grab their pinkie side with your left hand and move it diagonally towards the ground. This will be done in the same manner as "SPARROW HIT'S THE GROUND"

B. After bowing and locking the wrist, your right hand will let go completely. Going over the top of their arm with your right arm, you will swing low and turn your hips to the right. This will result in a rather severe arm lock if done correctly.

Cobra Leaves the Basket

This technique is against a two handed choke. You will put your hands together in a 'prayer' position. Leaning back slightly you will shoot your hands straight up between both of their arms. Moving your hands outwards, with your palms towards your face, you will strike both of your opponents arms, thus breaking or loosening their grip on your throat. Spreading your fingers, you will shoot your hands directly in towards their face. Like a snake biting its prey, you want to think of your fingers as fang's and strike the opponents eyes. Your hands will drop straight down, gripping both of your opponent's shoulders.

Your knee will lift high and hard, kneeing them in the groin. Turning your body slightly, you will rake your foot down hard on their kneecap. This is not meant to break their knee, rather bump or push hard enough to kick them away from you.

Bear Embraces the Sun

Against a two handed shoulder grab from the front. You will cross your arms on the inside of theirs, striking their inner forearms. Uncrossing your arms, you will push outwards hard, sliding their hands off of your shoulders.

A. After you have removed their hands from your shoulders, you will clamp your hands down hard on their shoulders and bring your knee upward, striking their groin. Turning your body slightly, you will rake your foot down hard on their kneecap. This is not meant to break their knee, rather bump or push hard enough to kick them away from you. Essentially, the A technique is exactly the same as the end of 'COBRA LEAVES THE BASKET'

B. After you have removed their hands from your shoulders, you will clamp both hands around the back of their head. Pulling their head downwards hard, you will raise your front knee at the same time, kneeing them in the face.

Dragon Wields a Mace

This is done from a single shoulder grab on your right side. Reaching across your body with your left hand, you will pin their hand to your shoulder. Stepping to your left side, you will stretch their body towards you, exposing the fold of their arm. Keeping them pinned, you will bring your right arm up your center line, and palm's facing you, and striking the fold of your opponents arm hard. When they bend at the arm, you will first spread your fingers and cobra strike into their eyes with your right hand. Landing your right hand on their shoulder, you will grip and step towards them with your left foot and do a solid palm strike to their face with your left hand. Grabbing the back of their head with your left hand, you will pull their head down hard. Lifting your left knee while you pull their head down, you will strike them in the face with your knee.

Spitting Cobra

This technique is against a two handed shirt grab. Doing a "U-Punch" you will strike them in the face with your left hand and in the gut with the right hand at the same time. Your left hand will drop, clamping their hands on your shirt. Your right hand will become a snake. Spreading your fingers, your right hand will go through the middle of their arms and strike them in the throat. Turning your hips and body to the right, you will squeeze your left elbow down over their hands to keep them in place. Your right arm will turn into a right outward block, creating a gap. Using that gap to your advantage, you will immediately strike their eyes with your right hand by spreading your fingers into a snake.

Chicken's Talon

This technique does technically have an A and a B. Although, the technique is the same whether it is against a straight across wrist grab or a cross wrist grab. I recommend always teaching and learning it from a straight across wrist grab. Once you have it down, try it against a cross wrist grab. As the opponent grab's your right wrist with their left hand (straight across), you will step back with your left foot and turn your hips. Your right hand will circle counter clockwise under their arm and grab their wrist. Pulling them towards you, your right foot will kick either their ribs or knee (depending on practitioner's height or flexibility). Stepping towards them with your left foot, you will bring your left hand in an upward thrust into the fold of your opponent's arm. (Think of how you would serve a volley ball underhanded). Once you have folded your opponents arm, you will immediately move your left hand onto your opponent's elbow. Now both hands should be on the outside of their arm and they should be in a "Chicken Wing" position. You ward off by sinking your weight into them and pushing them away.

Water Collides With Cliff

This technique is against a two handed wrist grab. You will bring both hand first up your center line, palms towards you. Then they will raise and go outward then sink and go outward. This entire motion should be ONE motion and to me resembles the shape of butterfly wings.)(This simple symbol should show the path of your hands. Once your hands have broken free, your right hand will throw a right hook to the face. Once contact has been made, you will turn your hip to the right and immediately strike them with a right back fist to the face followed directly by the ridge of your left palm hitting them in the chest, resulting in a hard push or ward off.

Evading the Sun

This is against an overhead club. If you do not have a bat or stick or anything blunt to practice with, a simple 'Chop' upon their head would work. As the club is coming down, you will step to your left and at the same time push their hand away with your left hand. This should be a push down in a motion from your left ear straight inward towards your nose. It may take some practice, but essentially, it is a push more than an awkward slap. Once you have stepped out of the path of the weapon and pushed, your right hand will come under your left on your opponent's arms. I use the term "normal body posture" here. Both hands should be on your opponents arm but they should not be crossed or uncomfortable. Adjust yourself so you are in a "normal body posture". Sinking your weight into them you should push them away from you.

Breaking the Cloud

This is against a right jab. Your left hand will be in front of your face in a defensive position. When the punch comes in, your left hand will slap it or redirect it away from your face by slapping it away from the outside of your opponent's fist. Immediately, your right fist will strike through your opponent's inner forearm, ending up on the outside of their arm. Your right hand will push down, followed by your left hand pushing down while you strike them in the face with a right back fist. Your right hand will drop and grab the opponents arm while your left elbow raises straight up into their outstretched elbow. The bump should be hard enough to jar the opponent. In severe cases, such as wielding a knife or being outnumbered, this should be hard enough to break their elbow. Once you have struck your opponent's elbow, both hands should drop to the outside of their arm in "natural posture position". Sinking your weight into them, you should push or ward off your opponent.

Catching the Koi

This technique is against a right jab. As the punch is coming in, with your left hand at a defensive position, you will slap or push their punch away from the outside of their fist. Your right fist will come up under their punch and strike them under the bicep. Turning your fist into an "eagle's beak" you will twist and strike them hard in the armpit with your knuckle. Stepping back with your left leg you will grip their arm as if it was a ball bat. Turning your hip as you rotate, you will swing or throw your opponent

Monkey Brushes its Hair

From the defensive position with your left hand in front of your face, you will slap the incoming punch with your left hand and bring your right hand upwards in an elbow thrust. This should be on the outside of the punch and look as if you are brushing your own hair. At the same time, you will take a large step forward with your right foot.

Turning your body, your right hand should just below or on your opponents nose and your left hand should go on the lower spine. Pushing down from the face and in from the spine should result in your opponent folding in half and hitting the ground.

Monkey Dance

This technique is from a shoulder grab from the back. You will place your right hand on your left shoulder pinning their hand. Stepping back with your left leg, (cross step behind right leg) you will use your left hand to chop your opponent's groin. Staying low, you will turn your hips, twirling your body underneath your opponent's arms and give an additional chop to the groin with your right hand. You should be facing your opponent at this point.

Left forearm will move to just above their hips and right hand will cup behind and just above their knee. Standing up, you will push down with your forearm and lift up with your right hand, resulting in a take down.

Repulse Monkey

At the defensive position with your left hand in front of your face, you will evade or slap your opponent's punch with your left hand. "Brushing your hair" you will step forward with your right leg and bring up your elbow on the outside of your opponents arm. You will turn your body and your hips so your left leg is behind your opponent's right knee.

Dropping your left elbow and squatting (keep back straight), you will place your elbow on your opponent's hips. With a hard push of the elbow in the direction of the ground you should drop your opponent.

Twirling the Sun

From the defensive position, with left hand in front of face you will come up your center-line and turn your hips. Catching your opponent's right punch on the inside with an "inward cloud hands", you will shoot your right hand to their right ear. Taking a step backwards, you will twirl their head underneath their own outstretched arm.

The result will be that you are behind them. If you were able to keep hold of their arm, this would automatically turned into a joint lock. On the occasion that you failed to hold on, end this technique with a choke hold.

Monkey Wields a Scimitar

From the defensive position with left hand in front of face, you will come up your center-line and catch their punch on the outside with your right hand. Immediately, your left hand will shoot up and "bump" their elbow. Sinking down and dropping your hands to the outside of their arm, you will finish up with "Repelling the cloud"

Five Sword's And a Spear

The movements on this technique is a little harder. This is one of those techniques you may need to spend extra time with your instructor to make it feel fluid.

From the defensive position, against a right hook, you will step into it with your right leg and both hands will block with a chopping motion on the inside of the punch. Though not perfect, essentially, your left hand should have blocked on one side of the fold of the arm, and your right hand should be on the other. Your right hand will chop their throat (1 count).

Your left hand will palm their face while the right hand moves to right hip. (2 count).

Your right hand will strike their ribs or gut with a hard upper cut style punch, while your left hand moves to your right shoulder. (3 count).

Your left hand will chop to their left throat or collar bone as your right hand rears back by your ear. (4 count).

Your right hand will chop the bridge of their nose as your left hand tucks underneath your right elbow (5 count).

Your left hand will shoot out in a hard palm strike, repelling or pushing your opponent away (spear).

Gorilla Pushes the Wall

In the defensive position with your left hand in front of your face, you will slap and grab your opponent's right hand with your left. Your right hand will hammer-fist your opponent's ribs. Pushing down on their hand and bringing your right hand above, you will back fist to the bridge of their nose. Dropping your right hand to their arm, you will grab and release with the left. Using a hard palm strike, you will strike their face with your left hand. Stepping to the side, you will stretch out their arm and push in on their face, dislocating their shoulder.

Sword Strikes Snake

At the defensive position with left hand in front of your face, against a right punch, you will turn your hips and bring your right hand up your center-line, catching the arm and holding on from the outside. Stepping with your left leg, you will shoot out your left arm underneath their elbow, pulling down and resulting in a break.

Stepping even, you will transfer their arm from your right hand to your left. Cross stepping your right leg over your left and then stepping your left leg back, you will drop your elbow into their ribs. Going under their arm, you will place your free hand on their shoulder and perform "wing break".

Drunk Twiddles Thumbs

This technique is against a clutching grab from the back. Dropping your hands down you will grab both thumbs and torque them until their grip breaks loose. Cross stepping with your left leg behind your right, you will duck under their arms and push forward into what we call the "stupid lock". This will their left arm over the top of their right arm in almost an x shape. Pushing down will take them to the ground, flip them, or break their arm. Depending on the speed and pressure.

Drunken Monkey

This technique is against a double punch. First a dominant right punch followed by a left punch. This would be useful in a drunken rumble or street fight where the opponent don't know much more than trying to swing wildly and over power you.

Stepping in and blocking a right punch with a two handed chop (five swords) on the INSIDE, you will step forward with your right leg and block with your left hand on the wrist side of the elbow and your right hand just outside of the fold of the elbow closer to the centerline of your opponent.

Left hand will chop to the throat, right hand will palm to the face. Your right hand will chamber on the right side. As the left punch is coming in, you will bring your hand up your centerline and turn your hips, catching the punch on the inside. Gripping their wrist with your right hand, you will C-shape your leg BEHIND their left foot. Sweeping their leg, you will push in on their center-line with a palm thrust to their chest with your left hand. This will take some practice and should be one fluid movement.

Swords on the Sun

Against a right punch, from the defensive position, you will come up your center-line with your right hand and turn your hips, catching the fist from the outside. You will grip the wrist with your right hand and smash their elbow with your left elbow. Your left hand will immediately palm strike to the face. The left hand will drop to grip the wrist as the right hand palm strikes the face. Stepping to the left slightly you will push and pull the pull strike so that the pressure is on the shoulder.

Cupping their head with your right hand, you will twirl them so their back is exposed. You will end the fight with either a kick to the knee or a rear naked choke. (Based on ability and instructor's advice).

Weaving the Basket

This technique is against a two handed shirt grab from the front. Take your right hand OVER their left hand and UNDER right hand. Staying close to their right wrist, you will turn your hips grip their right hand your right hand. Placing your left hand on their exposed right elbow, you will pull down with your right and raise their elbow with your left. This should result in a pretty nice joint lock.

Drunken Eagle

This technique technically has an A and a B but it's taught on one side. The same concepts will be mirrored for the opposite side. This is against a straight across shoulder grab on the left side. Cross stepping backwards, with your right foot in front of your left, you will repel their arm with a double chop. Your left fist will become an "eagles beak" and you will come up your centerline and strike their throat. At the SAME TIME, you will lift your right knee high into the air.

Turning your hips to the left, you will kick with your right leg, aiming for either knee cap or groin depending on your abilities.

Drunk Leans on Tree

This technique is against a two handed shoulder grab from behind. Leaning your weight backwards against them, you will cross step your left foot BEHIND your right foot. Ducking underneath their arms, you will grip their hand or wrists with your right hand and push down on their shoulder with the left. (Breaking Sparrow's Wings).

As they bend, you will slide down with your left hand and grip the outside of their thumb, resulting in a joint lock.

Saluting the Ball

This technique has an A and a B. The big difference is simply whether or not it is against a "straight across" wrist grab or a "cross handed" wrist grab.

    A.   From a "straight across" wrist grab (practiced on the right wrist) you will bring your right wrist straight up to your forehead on the outside of their arm. Turning your hips to the left, you will push in on their wrists. Once the contact is broken, you will grip their wrist with your right hand and turn hips to the right. Your Left hand will go OVER their arm and torque their elbow. This shall be a "energy ball"

    B.   Against a "cross grab" (practiced right side still) you will bring right hand up the centerline and turn hips to the right, gripping their wrist. Your left hand will go OVER their arm and rest on their elbow. In extreme cases, this can easily be turned into a break at your opponents elbow.

Enter Dan-Tien

This technique is against a one handed hammerlock practiced on the right side

As soon as you are put in a hammerlock, you will step FORWARD with your right leg, turning your hips to the right. At the SAME TIME, you will make your fingers sharp and strong, thrusting your right finger tips into their Dan Tien (belly button).

Turning your hips to the right, you will sink your right elbow and your body weight into their centerline. Bringing your right hand up your own centerline and turning, you will catch their wrist and grip.

Stepping with your left foot, you will end the technique with your left hand at their shoulder, performing "Sparrow Breaks It's Wings".

Gorilla Weaves the Basket

Against a two handed shirt grab, this technique will PUNCH in from both sides of their fists, immediately followed by a "U Punch". The left hand will punch the face and right will punch the stomach.

From there, your right hand will go OVER their left and UNDER their right. You will perform "Weaving the Basket" resulting in a joint lock.

Sword Strikes Sparrows Wing

From the defensive position, step forward with your left leg. Bringing your hands from ear to hip, you will first strike with the right hand, then immediately follow with the left hand. After two chops to the shoulder area, your left hand will pivot low, chopping the groin.

Your right hand will palm the face then turns to push the right side of your opponents head. Your left hand will push on the right shoulder.

This technique technically has a part B. However, it is the same movement but done with opposite hands on the opposite side. Practice both

The Five Gorillas

From the defensive position and against a right punch, you will step forward with your right leg. Using a "horizontal gunt" you will drive your right wrist through your opponents forearm. Gripping with opponent's wrist with your left hand, you will use your right hand to back fist the ribs. Pushing down with your left hand, you will bring your right fist over your opponent's arm and drive a back fist to the nose. Switching hands, you will grip the wrist with your right and back fist the nose with the left. From here, you will perform, Sun Beats Wall.

Lion Strikes Prey

From the defensive position, against a right punch, come up your center-line with your right hand, catching your opponent's right punch from the outside. Stepping forward with your left hand you will grab your opponent from BEHIND the head gripping their hair and pulling back. Hard palm strike to the nose with the right hand and raking down the face, starting with the eye sockets.

Holding the right side of their head with your left hand, you will bring your right elbow inward hard to their face.

The Snake and the Dart

From the defensive position, you will "slap" your opponent's fist from the outside. Making your finger and thumb into a 'gun' shape, you will poke your opponent in the eye. When the next punch comes in on the opposite side you will repeat the process. On the third punch, instead of making a gun, you will spread out all four fingers and strike hard to both eyes. This should be done as if your arm was the head of a snake and the fangs are blinding.

Yin Yang Sun

From a straight across wrist grab, you will turn your hips slightly to left, pushing your arm over the top of your opponents and bringing it back across your center-line in a "C-Shape". From there, you will turn your hips back to the right and continue to swing your arm. Your left hand will cover the opponents elbow. You should now have made an "energy ball". It will end with an arm lock on your right side.

Hammer Strikes Anvil

Against a single hand shirt grab, your
opposite fist will punch directly into the forearm or
wrist of your opponent. Swing hard and swing fast.
The impact will affect your opponents grip and their
hand should be cleared from your shirt.

Internal Concepts

When practicing Two Wolf Taijiquan, one must focus on BOTH the internal and external applications. Yes, there are some great self-defense applications in this system, but more than that, it is a whole body system. It helps the practitioner achieve a balance in their own self. We will train the body, the mind, and the spirit. Below is some of the basic concepts that shall be taught with the internal portion of Two Wolf.

~~*

Guided Meditation

In order to achieve focus and clarity, one must train the mind. In the beginning this can be achieved by forcing the mind to create and destroy a simple object. The goal here is not in the perfection of the technique as much as it is in achieving one simple objective. This objective consists of clearing the mind. Did the practitioner force the mind to follow his or her instructions? Were there any interruptions? Ideally, with a little bit of practice, this technique will be used to clear the mind completely before any deeper meditation practices are performed.

.

The Ball and the Chalkboard

Imagine a blank black chalkboard. On that chalkboard slowly draw a perfect circle starting from the top and slowly curving counter-clockwise. Once you have created the circle, reverse direction and erase the circle slowly in a clockwise direction.

Practice both drawing and erasing the circle until it is a smooth transition. Do this several times and eventually draw the circle and leave it on the chalkboard. Now visualize that chalk circle coming off of the board and hovering by itself. Spin the circle. First spin the circle slowly, then increase the speed of the spin. Slow. Fast. Slower. Keep complete control of the circle as you do this. Eventually make the circle stop completely and stay hovering in front of your mind's eye.

Now I want you to give the circle a third dimension. Make the circle into a bubble. Control the bubble with your mind. Make it dance and float in the wind. Back and forth and up and down. Get creative with the bubble. I want you to practice this until you have complete and utter control.

Now make the bubble land on the black chalkboard. It will pop and there will be nothing left except a blank chalkboard that is ready to be written on. Hold that image.

If this basic meditation exercise worked

properly. Your mind should be completely blank and ready to be trained. There should be no distracting thoughts or images cascading through the mind. There is nothing but a big black blank "chalkboard." You are now ready to take on a deeper meditation since you have achieved focus and control over your own muddy mind.

Chakra Meditation

The Seven Chakras
- Root Chakra
- Abdomen Chakra
- Solar Plexus Chakra
- Heart Chakra
- Throat Chakra
- Third Eye Chakra
- Crown Chakra

~~*

Chakra Meditation

Let us focus on healing the seven main chakras and clearing any energy blocks. We will replace them with positive thoughts and feelings. Find a comfortable spot or lie down and close your eyes. Begin to breathe very slowly and deeply. With each outward breath you are releasing any tensions that you may have. Start by becoming aware of the planet earth below you.

Imagine that there really is a connection between yourself and the earth. Visualize a beam of light that starts at the top of your head and moves downwards through your whole body. Imagine the beam of light coming out of the soles of your feet.

See the beam of light spreading out like the roots of a tree. Visualize these roots as they go deeper and deeper into the earth. Feel yourself going deeper and deeper into relaxation. Throughout the whole healing session you will continue feeling safe and secure as you know that you are grounded to the earth.

~~*

Start to become aware of the first energy center, the base chakra that is located at the base of your spine. This is related to the color red. It is also related to your sense of smell and your survival instinct.

Visualize this area at the base of your spine as being a rotating sphere of energy. A pulsating positive healing energy from the universe comes into your body and releases any blocked energy or negative emotions.

~~*

Now start to become aware of the second energy center located just below your navel known as the Abdomen Chakra. This is related to the color orange. It is related to your sense of taste. Visualize this center as a rotating energy sphere pulling in positive healing energy from the universe into your body and releasing old blocked energy and negative emotions that may be there.

Continue to visualize the color orange and feel yourself become connected with feelings of creativity, harmonious relationships, and balanced sexual energy.

~~*

Become aware of another energy area. This is the third or Solar Plexus chakra. It is located just above your navel but below your chest. This is related to the color yellow. It is related to your sense of sight. Visualize this as a rotating yellow sphere of energy, pulling positive energy from the universe into your body and releasing old blocked energy and negative emotions that may be there and replacing it with only positive energy. Continue to visualize the color yellow and as you do this focus on feelings of personal power, enhanced energy, and self- control.

~~*

Now start to become aware of the forth energy center known as the Heart chakra located in the center of your chest. This is related to the color green. It is related to your sense of touch and feelings of compassion and love. Visualize this as rotating sphere of green energy, pulling positive energy from the universe into your body and releasing old blocked energy and negative emotions that may be there. Continue to visualize the color green and as you do this focus on feelings of love and compassion towards all things.

~~*

Now start to become aware of the fifth

energy center known as the Throat chakra located in the center of your throat. This Throat chakra is related to the color blue and it is related to sound, speech, and communication. Visualize this as rotating sphere of blue energy, pulling positive energy from the universe into your body and releasing old blocked energy and negative emotions that may be there. Continue to visualize the color blue and as you do this focus on feelings of self-expression and communication.

~~*

Now start to become aware of the sixth energy center known as the Third Eye chakra located at the center of your forehead just above your eyes. This is related to the color indigo it is related to light and vision. Visualize this as a rotating sphere of indigo energy, pulling positive energy from the universe into your body and releasing old blocked energy and negative emotions that may be there. Continue to visualize the color indigo and focus on feelings of intuition and insight and being able to see everything clearly.

~~*

Now start to become aware of the seventh and final energy center often referred to as your Ground chakra. It is located at the very top of your head. This is related to the color violet it is related to thought, knowledge, and intuition. Visualize this as a rotating violet sphere, pulling positive energy from the universe into your body and releasing old blocked energy and negative emotions. Continue to visualize the color violet and start to feel yourself connecting to your higher self and feelings of wisdom.

~~*

Now visualize a line running through all seven chakras connecting them all together and bringing you a great feeling of balance and well-being. As you bring all the colors together, feel yourself being surrounded by an amazing Technicolor rainbow of glorious healing light. You have created a healing energy within your whole body which will continue to heal your body long after this session has ended.

Now visualize your chakras closing one at a time from your Base chakra to your Ground chakra and every chakra is now fully energized, healed, and balanced. You will continue to feel energized and totally uplifted for a long time. You will feel much more confident in all aspects of your life. You will feel more creative and will accept and love yourself as you are.

You find yourself being more and more compassionate towards others and loving towards yourself. The love you give out is multiplied and returned to you tenfold. You developed an incredible energy and you have succeeded in raising your vibration to a higher level. You will also find it much easier to express your thoughts and feelings. You have an amazingly strong self- belief. You are very intuitive and full of knowledge and wisdom. You will achieve great things now. You will be able to develop a greater understanding of life as you become more and more enlightened and aware as you continue to connect with this infinite power within yourself.

Five Element Breath

Relax, breathing your natural breath. As you do the breath pattern for each element in turn, attune with the cosmic element and experience its qualities within you. Experience the purification of your being on all levels: physical, mental, heart, soul, spirit. Perform five breaths for each element, or longer.

- **Earth**: *Inhale nose, exhale nose*
  Qualities: nurturing, solidity.
  Movement: spreading horizontally.
  Color: yellow-brown. Sense: touch
- **Water**: *Inhale nose, exhale mouth*
  Qualities: fluidity, purifying, giving life.
  Movement: downwards.
  Color: green. Sense: taste
- **Fire**: *Inhale mouth, exhale nose.*
  Qualities: enthusiasm, transmutation.
  Movement upward.
  Color: red. Sense: smell
- **Air**: *Inhale and exhale mouth*
  Qualities: freedom, releasing from constructs, cosmic identity.
  Movement zig-zag.
  Color: blue. Sense: hearing

- **Ether**: *Very fine breath inhaling and exhaling through the nose*
  Qualities: 'emotion of the soul'.
  Peace. Unity.
  Movement: stillness.
  Color: white. Sense: sight.

Five Organs Energy Breathing

The Five Organ Breathing Exercises are part of the Wu Dang style. This is a specialty style combining Taoist and Buddhist teachings with internal and external characteristics. The first part of Five Organ Breathing is an internal style which can be traced back to the master "Long Eyebrow" who lived at the beginning of the last century.

The Five Organ Breathing Exercise strengthens and energizes the major organ systems. There are five sounds: Xu (shew), Ke (kuh), Hu (who), Xia (shaw), and Chui (chwee) are used to strengthen the liver, heart, spleen, lungs, and kidneys. The sound and the shape of the mouth stimulate the acupuncture points which influence these five organs. Sick energy is expelled and the organs are energized.

~~*

Startup

Breathe six times, bend slightly forward. Relax the shoulders, waist, knees, and ankles. Inhale through the nose and exhale through the mouth. While inhaling, raise the hands, palm down, up to the shoulders. Swing the arms open, hold your breath briefly. Now lower the arms, palms down, and exhale. Repeat six times.

Liver Breathing

The liver is governed by the element wood, and produced by the element water. The sound for the liver exercise is Xu (pronounced shew). The shape of the mouth is like an exaggerated smile with the corners turned up. The sound resonates in the throat creating a vibration with the natural frequency to stimulate liver functions.

Close the eyes. Raise the arms, palms up, inhale and visualize vital, fresh Qi entering the toes and traveling to the middle Dan Tien–in the center of your chest. Hold your breath for a few seconds while the Qi circulates, then exhale making the "Xu" sound as your hands descend. Visualize sick Qi traveling out through the arms and leaving your body through the center of the palms. Open your eyes widely during exhalation. This is the only time the eyes are opened during the Five Organ Breathing Exercises. It is important not to look at anyone; sick Qi also leaves through the eyes and can be harmful.

~~*

Heart Breathing

This exercise is for the heart and circulatory system. The heart is governed by the element fire, which is produced by the element wood. The sound for the heart exercise is Ke (Kuh). When making the "Ke" sound, press the tip of the tongue slightly behind the lower teeth.

Inhale, raise the arms and direct the Qi from your big toes to the middle Dan Tien–in the middle of your chest. Hold your breath and rotate the hands quickly, and raise them above the head. Visualize Qi circulating throughout the body. If you have high blood pressure, don't reach quite so high.

Point the hands together when exhaling and make the "Ke" sound. Exhale and visualize the qi traveling from the middle Dan Tien through the arms and out the tips of the middle fingers. Relax your body as the arms descend.

~~*

Spleen Breathing

This exercise if for the Spleen and digestive system. The spleen is governed by the element earth, which is produced by the element fire. The sound is Hu (who). The mouth should be round, like a monkey's with the tongue slightly rolled up.

As you inhale, visualize Qi rising from the big toes to the middle Dan Tien–in the middle of your chest. Exhale and visualize it going through the arms and out the center of the palms. Start by holding the Qi ball in from of your abdomen. Rotate the hands. One arms extends upward with the palm up toward heaven, and the other downward connecting to the earth Qi. The upper arm should fully extend, stretching the stomach on first one side then the other, which improves digestion.

~~*

Lung Breathing

The Lungs are governed by the element metal, produced by the element earth. The sound for the lungs is Xia (shaw). The mouth is opened wide, softly projecting the sound and letting it end abruptly. The eyes should be closed while the Qi circulates in the body. Inhale, visualizing the Qi rising from the toes to the middle Dan Tien–in the middle of your chest. When exhaling, visualize it flowing from the mid-chest point through the arms and out the center of your palms. The "Xia" sound expels harmful Qi from the lungs.

Start by raising the hand, palms up and fingers pointed toward each other. Raise the hands to the middle Dan Tien. Hold the breath until the hands have reached the edge of your shoulders, turning the palms out. Let the qi circulate while you are holding your breath. Exhale, making the "Xia" sound, and turn the palms out.

~~*

Kidney Breathing

The Kidneys are governed by the element water, which is produced by the element metal. The sound for the kidney is Chui (chwee). To make the sound, the mouth protrudes a little while raising the tongue slightly. Make the sound just loud enough to hear and feel it.

To begin the exercise, rub the kidney area with the back of the hands while inhaling. In this exercise, the Qi is directed up from the bubbling well point, located just behind the ball of each foot. Hold the breath while bringing the hands to the front with fingers pointed toward each other and palms facing you. Keep the hands in this position as you exhale, while bring the arms down and bending the knees.

~~*

Triple Burner Breathing

The sound for the Triple Burner is Shee. Inhale, raising the hands to the mid-chest, palms facing you. Rotate the hands quickly, while holding your breath. Raise the hands above the head. Turn the palms inward, and skim your hands down your face and then down your body. Continue down the rib cage and down to the knee. Brush the sick, stagnant Qi away from your body quickly. Visualize

Qi rising from the big toes to the middle Dan Tien–in the middle of your chest–during the inhale, then going out through the arms and the center of your palms during the exhale.

You won't find the Triple Burner as an organ in Western medicine. However, according to the Chinese, it directly affects the body's overall metabolism and plays and important part in regulating the body's entire energy field.

~~*

Closing

Rub your hands together until they are warm. Rub your face vigorously, then rub your eyes, your nose, and any wrinkles. Comb the hair with the fingertips, firmly stimulating the scalp. The fingers carry Qi to the acupuncture points on the head, which are connected to the body's nervous system. Now massage the ears. Pull down on the earlobes from the top to the bottom. Next pat the head in rotation. Start gently and increase the force. This prevents a build- up of Qi in the head. Pat the front of your body from the chest down to the ankles. Then do each arm, starting close to the body and working outward. Finally pat down the left and right side of the under arm. This is to keep the Qi from setting in one part of the body and make it return to the Dan Tien–in the middle of your chest.

Now pat the kidneys with the back of the hands. This stimulates the adrenal glands, which rest on top of each kidney.

Exercise the Qi ball. Push and pull the Qi. Circulate it around the body, harmonizing Yin and Yang energy. When pulling the hands apart, there should be a force holding them together. When pushing, there should be a resistance. The motion should be small and slow as if holding a big balloon. Visualize the qi being generated. Your palms may feel one or more of eight sensations: soreness, numbness, swelling, cold, hot, aching, itching, or the passing of a breeze.

This completes the Five Organ Breathing exercise. It is best to do the complete series in the correct order. Each of the exercises should be done in multiples of six. If you have weakness in one organ, you can spend more time on that one, but the whole series should be completed each time you practice.

Pushing Hands

Just like all Tai Chi systems, Two Wolf Taijiquan uses Pushing Hands to help train the practitioner in the external and internal connection between the martial arts. We use it for sensitivity training and as a stepping stone for our own unique method called "Wolf's Den"

"In Tai Chi, pushing hands is used to acquaint students with the principles of what are known as the "Eight Gates and Five Steps," eight different leverage applications in the arms accompanied by footwork in a range of motion, intended to allow students to defend themselves calmly and competently if attacked. Also known as the "13 original movements of tai chi", a posture expressing each one of these aspects is found in all tai chi styles. Training and pushing hands competitions generally involve contact but no strikes.

The three primary principles of movement cultivated by push hands practice are:

- Rooting - Stability of stance, a highly trained sense of balance in the face of force.
- Yielding - The ability to flow with incoming force from any angle. The practitioner moves with the attacker's force fluidly without compromising their own balance.

- Release of Power (Fa Jing) - The application of power to an opponent. Even while applying force in push hands one maintains the principles of Yielding and rooting at all times."

-Wikipedia-

No matter how or who attempts to define what Pushing Hands really is, it is a very important tool and is something that needs to be learned, practiced, felt, and utilized for a deeper understanding of Tai Chi.

Wolf's Den

This is unique to this system. Two people will stand in a small circle with their hands touching just like in "Pushing Hands". Utilizing the same concepts, they will go beyond and demonstrate their rooting and yielding with joint locks. This practice is more about strategy and "feeling" where the next movement is more than it is about power.

Taking turns, one person will place the other person in a lock of their choice. Their goal: to knock the other off balance and get their palm to touch the ground OR make the other person step out of the ring.

We practice this so that if you are grabbed by anyone in any manner in a real life situation, you will simply react and escape with your life.

Wolf's Den is NOT a replacement for Pushing Hands. It is simply the YANG to its YIN. It is slightly more aggressive, but holds true to the same principles. A good practitioner will never value one practice over the other, but rather understand and practice both and gain the experience and knowledge they both have to offer.

Path Walker

In many Martial Arts they have a structured system full of ranks and titles. I do see the necessity for this, but disagree with it. I do not believe anyone can "master" a martial art. There will be so much to improve on, so much to learn. You can go through the motions and understand the techniques. You can be wise and have a deep understanding of everything involved.

What you cannot do is know all that there is to know and know it perfectly. A path walker is a term that is used referring to anyone in Two Wolf that has the life experience and practice to lead others down the path of self-improvement and discipline.

They have not "mastered" anything. They have simply decided to keep walking this path and keep trying to improve. Besides gaining the knowledge of everything the Two Wolf system has to offer, a great path walker is someone who has, or has decided to dedicate themselves to achieving several life traits as well.

Listing positive attributes would be mundane and irrelevant seeing that there are so many truly positive gifts to mankind. However, here are a few qualities a good path walker should try to possess.

- **_Right Thought:_** One should always attempt to think only happy and positive thoughts about themselves and others. Too much negativity will block the Chakras and muddy up the soul. Never think the worst about someone and always believe they have good intentions.
- **_Right Speech:_** One should analyze their thoughts before letting it materialize into words. What you say to people or about people matters. One simple negative phrase or misunderstanding can grow like a weed and choke out the natural beauty of the world. A good path walker will know when to hold their tongue and always trust themselves to speak only truth, _no matter the consequences_
- **_Humility:_** Even if you have achieved much in life, life has a way of making you understand that everything you have achieved in the material world does not matter. Be polite. Be happy. Most importantly, be your naked self. We all breathe, we all have needs and wants. You are equal to every man and woman that walks the earth.
- **_Poverty:_** This quality is the most

misunderstood. I am not saying to be poor. I am saying to place very little importance on how much money you have or how much money you can get. NEVER turn your back on someone in need just because they cannot pay you or there is nothing in it for you. Bottom line: *It is what you do with the money you have that matters.*

~~*

I hope this brief manual has inspired you to practice daily and you have a more thorough understanding of the Yin and Yang of Two Wolf Taijiquan.
For more information on this new unique style, feel free to contact me.

codytoye@gmail.com